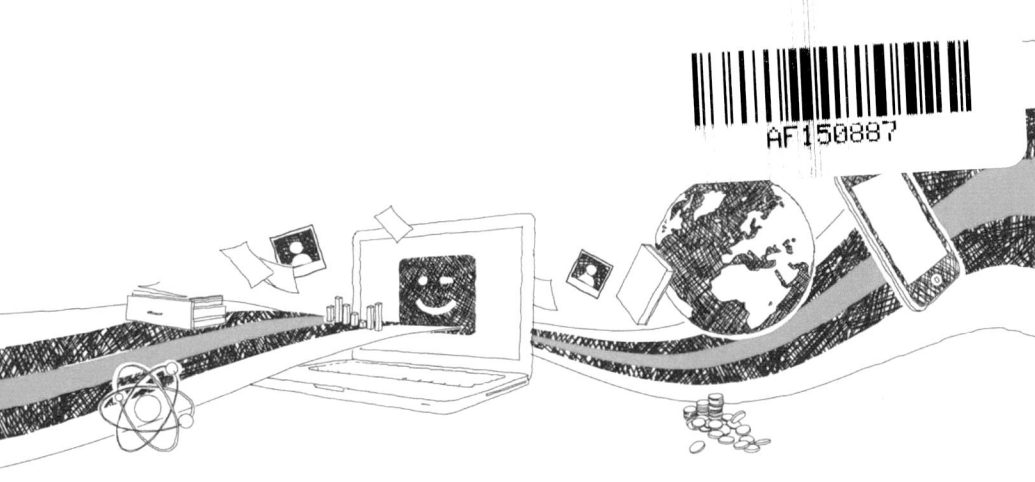
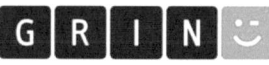

Bibliographic information published by the German National Library:

The German National Library lists this publication in the National Bibliography; detailed bibliographic data are available on the Internet at http://dnb.dnb.de .

Imprint:

Copyright © 2016 GRIN Verlag, Open Publishing GmbH
Print and binding: Books on Demand GmbH, Norderstedt Germany
ISBN: 9783668576735

This book at GRIN:

http://www.grin.com/en/e-book/381244/healthcare-industry-in-america-and-canada

Patrick Kimuyu

Healthcare Industry in America and Canada

GRIN Publishing

Healthcare Industry in America and Canada

Name: Patrick K. Kimuyu

Content

Introduction

Healthcare industry in America and Canada is believed to be one of the most sophisticated healthcare systems in the world, primarily in regard to healthcare sustainability and life expectancy of their populations. Thummalapally et al. (2013) reports "the United States has the largest healthcare services market in the world, representing a significant portion of the U.S. economy" (par. 2).

2

Ordinarily, healthcare systems in the U.S and Canada are experiencing related challenges. For instance, both systems are faced with an enormous public health challenges owing to the high incidence rates of non-communicable diseases such as obesity and its related health conditions which have increased the disease burden on healthcare systems. As a result, healthcare expenditure in the U.S and Canada has more than doubled in the past two decades owing to the unprecedented increase of healthcare costs (Douketis et al., 2007). It is reported that an estimated population of 97 million adults, in the U.S, are obese, and these statistics imply that the U.S healthcare industry is faced with immense challenges. On the other hand, Canada faces enormous challenges in healthcare delivery owing to the disease burden caused by non-communicable diseases. Makarenko (2010) remarks "in Canada, one issue that tends to prevail, arguably more than any other in Canadian public policy debate, is the issue of health care and health care delivery" (par. 1).

However, healthcare industry in the U.S and Canada differ significantly in terms of the forms of healthcare systems, styles of rationing healthcare, healthcare coverage and healthcare technologies adopted in the healthcare systems. Moreover, healthcare industry in the U.S and Canada manifest differences in regard to their impacts on the economy and healthcare policy reforms. Therefore, this research paper will provide an overview of the healthcare industry in the U.S and Canada. It will also provide a discussion on different aspects of these two healthcare systems, primarily with regard to the cost of healthcare in the two countries.

Health Systems

Healthcare systems adopted by the U.S and Canada are quite different in terms of government involvement in funding healthcare services. In Canada, healthcare industry is characterized by the adoption of a single-payer system in which the government is involved in all

3

healthcare funding. As a result, the Canadian population does not incur excessive costs in financing healthcare services although the private healthcare sector plays a pivotal role in healthcare service provision (Reinhardt, 2007). On the other hand, the U.S healthcare industry is characterized by a consumer driven healthcare system in which the government provides limited healthcare funding while consumers contribute the highest percentage of funding.

Canadian Single-Payer System

In regard to healthcare systems, the Canadian healthcare industry is characterized by a single-payer system of financing in which the government adopts a federalized system of funding. Mendelson (2010) observes "If the Canadian health-care system were a corporation, it would be among the biggest in the world" (par. 1). In this system, the Canadian government funds the largest percentage of healthcare costs although private enterprises act as the leading service providers. It is believed that, the Canadian's single-payer system has enabled the healthcare industry to realize remarkable growth and development in the past decade in which healthcare costs are believed to have decreased significantly owing to the benefits of the single-payer system.

In general, the Canadian single-payer healthcare system comprises of thirteen tax-financed health insurance systems which operate at the provincial level under the guidelines of the federal government based in Ottawa. It is believed that these guidelines enhance uniformity in the entire healthcare industry through facilitating cost sharing mechanisms within the single-payer system. For instance, the tax-financed insurance system at the provincial level provides healthcare services to the public and caters for the procurement of physician services under the platform of not-for-profit and for-profit delivery in which the single-payer system ensures efficient negotiations with healthcare providers on behalf on the customers (Reinhardt, 2007).

4

From a cost perspective, the single-payer healthcare system adopted by Canadian government encompasses several benefits, which are believed to have contributed significantly to the increase of life expectancy among the Canadian population. Single-payer systems are usually designed on the approaches of free-market environment; thus, uniformity is guaranteed. Reinhardt (2007) states "by virtue of their administrative simplicity, single-payer systems are the ideal platforms for uniform information infra - structure, based on common nomenclature and technical processes" (p. 40). The second benefit of the single-payer healthcare system is that the administrative cost of healthcare operations is relatively low compared to market oriented systems. This explains the reason, as to why, the Canadian healthcare industry is highly flexible and cost effective compared to the U.S healthcare industry which is based on the consumer market. Therefore, private insurers in Canada do not incur enormous costs on marketing, administration and profits because the single-payer system reduces healthcare operation costs (Reinhardt, 2007). It is also reported that a single-payer healthcare system seems the most appropriate for an egalitarian distribution ethic observed in healthcare. Therefore, Canadian population enjoys healthcare more as a right than a basic necessity of well-being.

U.S Consumer-Driven Healthcare

On the other hand, the U.S healthcare industry is based on the platform of market-oriented service delivery in which consumers contribute the highest percentage of healthcare funding. In consumer-driven healthcare system of the U.S, private healthcare providers and health insurance agencies engage in direct negotiations with consumers, and the government does not enter into negotiations with healthcare service providers on behalf of consumers. This is a significant contrast to the Canadian single-payer system where the government assumes the responsibility of making negotiations with healthcare providers on behalf of the consumers (Reinhardt, 2007).

Ideally, the U.S market-oriented healthcare system requires the beneficiaries of medicare and Medicaid health insurance plans to be subjected to a so-called high deductible health plan. This enables financial shifts from healthcare insurance agencies to consumers. As such, consumers have the greatest responsibility in financing healthcare systems in the U.S. it is believed that the universal healthcare strategy will enhance the consumer-driven healthcare to ensure that the U.S government does not carry the burden of healthcare costs.

Despite the benefits associated with a market-oriented healthcare system such as the reduction of government spending on healthcare services, this system causes significant disadvantages to health insurance providers and consumers. For instance, health insurance providers incur high administrative costs on markets and profits whereas consumers are exposed to exploitation by healthcare providers because the system is based on imperialism. In other words, benefits obtained from a monopolistic form of market environment are entirely absent because the U.S government allows private health insurance agencies to compete in the market-oriented system (Reinhardt, 2007). This phenomenon makes the U.S healthcare industry relatively different from the Canadian single-payer system because government monopoly is the principal feature of the Canadian healthcare industry.

Cost of Healthcare

Cost of healthcare in the U.S and Canadian healthcare industries is relatively different owing to the system adopted by each country. Ordinarily, Canada incurs low cost of healthcare compared to the U.S because its healthcare industry is stable and uniform; thus, it lowers the administrative cost of healthcare. In regard to the government spending, the U.S government spends heavily in healthcare compared to Canada and yet the latter covers all healthcare costs in its system. It is surprising to learn that Canada spent $2,120, in 2004, to cover all healthcare costs for its population far below the amount of money which was spent by the U.S government to finance half of the total healthcare costs for its population. In 2004, the U.S government spent $2,724 in healthcare costs despite the high consumer contribution for healthcare services. In general, Canadian government spent 9.8 percent of its GDP while the U.S spent 15.4 percent of its GDP although it experiences reduced healthcare responsibilities because half of the cost burden is placed on the consumers.

Styles of Rationing Healthcare

It is also believed that the healthcare industry in the U.S and Canada exhibits different trends in price rationing. In the U.S healthcare system, price rationing is capitalized because healthcare serves as one of the scarce resources (Reinhardt, 2007). Therefore, the U.S healthcare industry incurs hidden cost leading to unprecedented lost of value, primarily through the uninsured Americans who are estimated to be 39 million although the current healthcare reforms which aim at providing universal healthcare to all U.S citizens may address this issue (Shi & Singh, 2011). As a result, Americans incur immense out-of-pocket costs to cover their healthcare services. On the other hand, Americans who are insured are subjected to high insurance premiums to cater for the deficit caused by hidden costs.

In contrast, the egalitarian ethic of Canadian healthcare ensures all Canadians receive adequate healthcare services through the government-funded system. Therefore, healthcare is not regarded as a scarce resource which may attract price rationing. Instead, Canadians receive healthcare as a right, and they are not subjected to high tax-deductibles (Bercaw, 2011).

Coverage and Access to Healthcare

Coverage and access to healthcare is believed to be another significant factor which distinguishes healthcare industry in the U.S and Canada. In the U.S, universal healthcare has become a guarantee to special groups who are covered with medicare and Medicaid healthcare programs which are funded through tax-deductions from the employed U.S citizens. However, healthcare coverage and access is determined the concerned healthcare plans; either government-funded health insurance which accounts for only 27% or private health insurance plans.

Healthcare Technology

In regard to healthcare technology, both the U.S and Canadian healthcare industries seem to have capitalized on information technology to enhance healthcare service delivery and customer satisfaction. Tiwari (2013) reports "U.S and Canada lead healthcare IT outsourcing market 2018 forecasts in new research report" (par. 1). This approach is believed to have caused significant impacts on the U.S and Canadian economy. However, health outcomes remain different between the U.S and Canada in which Canadians are believed to be healthier compared to Americans.

Conclusion

In a brief conclusion, healthcare industry in the U.S and Canada is characterized with IT outsourcing and improved healthcare coverage and access. This is probably the reason as to why these two countries have the best healthcare systems in the world. However, it is worth noting that U.S uses a consumer-driven healthcare in which it covers half of healthcare costs whereas Canada uses a single-payer system with full government funding.

Despite the benefits associated with the U.S market-oriented healthcare, some people feel "The U.S. health care system is a giant money making scam that is designed to drain as much money as possible out of their pockets" (Snyder, 2013 par. 1). On the other hand, Canadian healthcare industry seems to be advancing in developing strategic healthcare plans to meet the current and future healthcare challenges (Bitti, 2012).

References

Bercaw, R. (2011). *Taking Improvement from the Assembly Line to Healthcare: The Application of Lean within the Healthcare Industry*. Boca Raton, FL: CRC Press.

Bitti, M. (2012). *A Remedial Strategy for Canada's Changing Healthcare Industry*. Retrieved from http://business.financialpost.com/2012/08/21/a-remedial-strategy-for-canadas-changing-healthcare-industry/

Douketis, J. et al. (2007). *2006 Canadian Clinical Practice Guidelines on the Management and Prevention of Obesity in Adults and Children*. CMAJ, 176(8):1–117. Retrieved from http://www.cmaj.ca/content/suppl/2007/09/04/176.8.S1.DC1/obesity-lau-onlineNEW.pdf

Makarenko, J. (2010). *Canada's Health Care System: An Overview of Public and Private Participation*. Retrieved from http://mapleleafweb.com/features/canada-s-health-care-system-overview-public-and-private-participation

Mendelson, R. (2010). *The worst-run industry in Canada: Health care*. Retrieved from http://www.canadianbusiness.com/business-strategy/the-worst-run-industry-in-canada-health-care/

Reinhardt, U. (2007). *Keeping Afloat the United States versus Canada*. Retrieved from http://www.princeton.edu/~reinhard/pdfs/MILKEN%20REVIEW%20CANADA%20vs%20US.pdf

Shi, L. & Singh, D. (2011). *Delivering Health Care in America*. Burlington, MA: Jones & Bartlett Publishers.

Snyder, M. (2013). *50 Signs That The U.S. Health Care System Is A Gigantic Money Making Scam*. Retrieved from http://theeconomiccollapseblog.com/archives/50-signs-that-the-u-s-health-care-system-is-a-gigantic-money-making-scam-that-is-about-to-collapse

Thummalapally, V. et al. (2013). *The Health and Medical Technology Industry in the United States*. Retrieved from http://selectusa.commerce.gov/industry-snapshots/health-and-medical-technology-industry-united-states

Tiwari, P. (2013). *US & Canada Lead Healthcare IT Outsourcing Market 2018 Forecasts in New Research Report.* Retrieved from http://www.prweb.com/releases/global-healthcare-it/outsourcing-market-report/prweb10996271.htm

YOUR KNOWLEDGE HAS VALUE

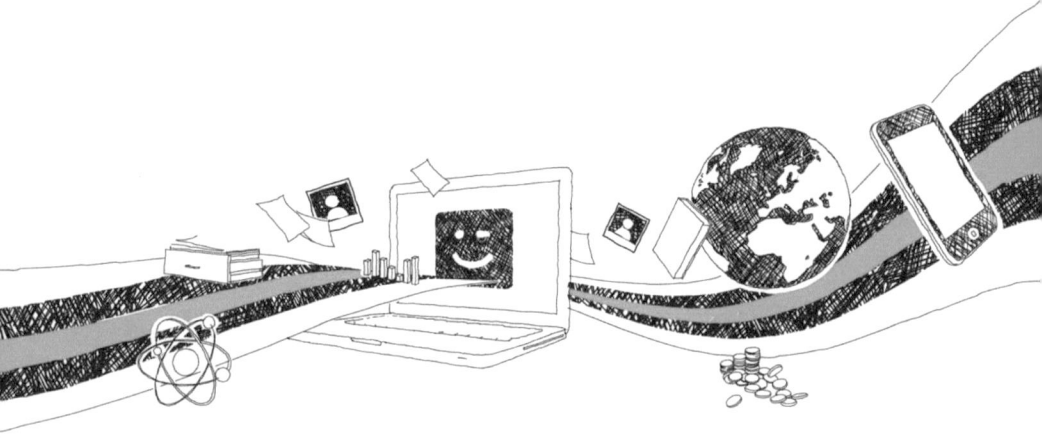

- We will publish your bachelor's and
  master's thesis, essays and papers

- Your own eBook and book -
  sold worldwide in all relevant shops

- Earn money with each sale

Upload your text at www.GRIN.com
and publish for free

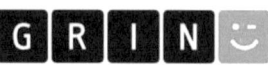